Dr. Farrah's Book of Nature and Alzheimer's Disease

By
Farrah-Arsenia Agustin-Bunch, MD

Disclaimer

This book is for educational and entertainment use only. Whatever information you gather in this literature you feel you want to utilize for your health or those associated with you, you are encouraged to ask your medical health professional.

Dr. Farrah does not offer any health advice or recommendation. Some of the information or articles presented here may need to be corrected and should be used responsibly. It is vital to refer to the references outlined in this book to ascertain their truthfulness.

If you are having a medical emergency, please stop reading this book and go to the nearest hospital or healthcare provider.

Contents

Introduction

The perfect introduction to this book is to tell the story of my friend who is afflicted with Alzheimer's disease.

P.A., 80 years old, female, married, has six children, is a licensed nurse, and worked for the state for 40 years before retiring. She usually helped care for her grandchildren and dogs during her retirement period. She also spent most of her time watching television shows. She was not sociable, preferring to stay in the house most of the time. Her diet was terrible. She lived on sugary and processed food as she had not cooked for her and her husband for decades. She lived in social isolation for years.

Her present condition started around three years ago when her children noticed some changes in her attitude and demeanor. She would suddenly become easily agitated and angered by minor, unreasonable incidents. She became hostile for no apparent reason. She would wander alone during the night outside her house and walk for hours until some neighbors would spot her and call the police. When in the house, P.A. would shop incessantly on the TV shopping network, buying things she does not need. Through the years, she accumulated useless objects and started hoarding them. Her home was filled to the ceiling, primarily with tissues, unwashed clothes, and plastic bags. As she became more socially withdrawn from her family and friends, she exhibited delusions toward her husband. P. A would accuse him of being a philanderer. "He is always running around with girls. He leaves me alone all the time!" She would also accuse him of taking her money, not feeding her, and being physically and verbally abusive to her. P.A.'s hygiene became so bad that she did not bathe for three months and would not change her clothes for a week or more. As her behavior worsened, her memory and recall became terrible, too. She would lose her dentures, cellphones, intimates, and shoes. In time, she has forgotten how to read and write. She would mumble words, talk incoherently, forget to use the proper word for a particular object, be unable to calculate simple math and fail to count and recite the alphabet. She stopped driving after nearly 60 years of experience. At this time, she would stay awake during the night and would sleep during the day. She refuses to eat and thus lost significant weight. When asked why, she would say, "My husband is poisoning me." Due to the persistence of these conditions, the family sought a neurologist's consultation. The doctor asked P.A. specific questions about her family and identity during the examination. She was unable to answer all of them. An MRI was requested, including a blood test. Blood sugar is high, while MRI results showed brain atrophy and ischemic strokes. The medical professional gave the grim diagnosis of Alzheimer's disease and vascular dementia. She was placed on antidepressants and memantine. None of the drugs helped alleviate her deteriorating cognition and behavior. P.A.'s condition worsened. The family had no recourse but to institutionalize her.

I wish to tell you that through professional help, there was a glimpse of hope in this terrible ordeal, but P.A.'s condition went downhill from there. She became incontinent, requiring multiple diaper changes. She was unable to bathe herself. She needs assistance with simple daily tasks. She would get lost in the halls of the home. She has not regained her appetite. She cannot remember her children and husband anymore. P. A. has no memory of the past or pleasure in anything.

Alzheimer's disease is a heartbreaking illness. It has no cure to date. The treatment available is to alleviate some symptoms. It is indeed a debilitating illness, a menace not only in the family, society, and the health care system. P.A.'s story is sad, but she is not alone. The global prevalence of this disease is staggering and is estimated to increase in the coming years. The burden of dementia is genuinely alarming.

What can we do? How can we stop this illness from the root? If Alzheimer's disease has no cure, what is the purpose of this book?

In this book, I will enumerate the modifiable risk factors that can be altered, how having the genetic predisposition doesn't predestine someone, and discuss the natural remedies that may help mitigate the occurrence or alleviate symptoms of Alzheimer's disease.

I pray that my readers will enjoy and learn from this book, which I enjoyed writing myself. I dedicate it to my husband, John, and my beautiful children, Kyla, Gabby, Henry, Duke, and Daisy.

Chapter 1
What is Cognitive Decline in the Elderly?

How often do you hear from an older adult that they struggle to remember the names of colleagues? Or do they need to remember where they placed the car keys? Noticeable changes in memory and slowing down in sensory perception may be expected in older adults.

But why does age-related cognition decline essential to identify? What sets dementia and average age-related memory loss apart?

A properly operating nervous system is necessary for an individual to function independently, drive safely, care for themselves, manage their assets, and make wise judgments. The ability and inability to perform daily activities equate to disability, which is not the same as aging.

Memory loss can be devastating for some. Many people have routines in place to preserve their executive functioning. My father used to write, while my grandfather believed that veganism helped him maintain his mental faculties.

What about you? What have you done thus far to protect your brain from natural degeneration or to slow down the inevitable?

Memory loss is scary and comical to many. I sometimes miss the names of my children. I asked my 182k Facebook followers for their funniest "lapse of memory" stories. These are the most hilarious comments I got.

"I was looking incessantly for my phone, and after a minute, I realized I already have them in my hand."

Katherine Gamboa

"When I went to the grocery on a single motorcycle, I arrived home on my commute. I realized that I left my motorbike. It is too much stress!"

Ja Alonzo

"I'm looking for my eyeglasses to find out later that I am wearing them!"

Nolie Tejada

"One time, when my kids were still young, my husband carried my daughter while looking after my son. Then suddenly he went looking for my daughter. He came up to me and kept asking where she was. I pointed out that he was carrying her."

Sanibel Daepo Yu

"I was looking for my medical file on my way to the doctor's clinic. I panicked because I thought I had left it somewhere. Then suddenly, my daughter said it's in your hand, Mom."

Janet Hechanova

"I was checking exam papers when somebody got a perfect score. I was delighted. But the test paper with the perfect score had no name! It took me a while to realize it was the answer key."

Aldeheid Heidi Angeles

"While eating lunch with my kids, we had some chit-chat. I was supposed to dip my chicken in its sauce, but since I got carried away by what we talked about, I dipped the glass with Coke on it."

Len Marollano

"Left the remote control in the fridge."

Jing Rol

"As I was riding a tricycle on my way home, I called my husband and informed him I was on my way. Then suddenly I realized that my phone was not in my bag. I panicked and started to worry that my phone was lost. My husband, who was in the line, said what phone are you talking about? Is that the phone you are using now?"

Chris Tine

"Just now, I thought I would shower at 4 pm, forgetting that I had already taken a shower at 8:30 am."

Jaz Rios

"I have been looking for my phone everywhere, only to find out it was in my armpit all along."

Maureen Michelle

"I once walked into a room and forgot why I was there. I went back to where I started to remember. It turns out I was looking for my keys, which were in my hand the whole time."

Shiela Salagubang

"I hurriedly came to my classroom and scolded all the students in that section. I reprimanded them for not cleaning their room and how to properly behave while waiting for their next teacher. Suddenly, I realized their faces were unfamiliar. I went to the wrong classroom."

Nits Stin

"I used an umbrella inside the mall. Then I caught myself in the big mirror."

Gnzn Mel

Temporary memory losses are not funny, but the stories of my followers are.

A person at an advanced age may experience minor or significant changes in their sensory perception, such as audition, olfaction, gustatory, and vision. These degenerative changes are regular and may result from nerve cell deaths. For example, my grandfather, who died at the age of 96, was half deaf and half blind. He also became selective with his food and, as a result, lost a lot of weight.

My father used to do many things at once. He was a salesman and juggled work and family life all the time. He was vibrant and had the energy for parties, recreation, and socialization. As he approached old age, his energy tanked. He would often sit in one place and struggle to perform three or two tasks simultaneously, which is common in the aging population.

There is a noticeable slowing down of information processing in the brain, which can be attributed to some alteration in the neuronal structures and their synapses. This can be evident through their language use, whether verbal, written, or nonverbal communication and motor activities. It takes time to name objects, people, and places. Memories are more complex than they used to be, so they struggle to tell stories. The accuracy of these stories may be in question. Their handwriting changes, making it less legible in time.

Communication and experiential skills, judgment and reasoning, knowledge, and behavior may or may not be slightly affected, but they are well preserved otherwise.

Typical age-related changes in the brain were studied with the use of MRI. The scientists noticed a decrease in the volume of the brain, which is restricted to some regions. Some neurons have a noticeable decline in number, dendritic spines, and axonic structures are altered, demyelination is apparent, and increased synaptic dysfunctions occur. These changes reflect the cognitive decline among older adults. This can be the reason why some older individuals often experience memory loss.

In addition, diabetes, hypertension, cardiovascular disease, cerebrovascular disease, and other chronic illnesses may contribute to the decline in the mental faculties of the aged. Also, inflammation, hypoxic episodes, and trauma can exacerbate the insult in the nervous system. Some psychological issues, such as depression, anxiety, and social isolation, may also wreak havoc on an already burdened brain. It is, therefore, essential to remain fit by adopting a healthy lifestyle, exercising, avoiding smoking, illicit drugs, and alcohol, and eating a well-balanced diet rich in plant-based foods, fibers, antioxidants, and essential fatty acids. Consumption of sugary, processed, and highly oxidized food should be kept at a minimum if none. Staying busy through socialization, maintaining a hobby, and engaging in mentally enhancing work or activities is also recommended. Meditation, laughter, optimism despite challenges, and peace with one's inner self and neighbors are essential throughout our lives.

Aging is normal, but it does not have to be painful or cumbersome for you, your family, or your friends. After all, aging is a privilege that is denied to the young. An older person can be functional in the later years of his life. Cognitive decline should not be a death sentence.

How can an older person remain engaged? What are the many ways he can do to stay "mentally in control"?

I asked on social media how people care for their aging brains. Here are the answers I got.

1. Answering word puzzles
2. Reading and memorizing Scriptures

3. Regular intake of food supplements, vitamins, and mineral and herbal supplements.
4. Exercise such as walking and dancing.
5. Optimism and kindness
6. Eating healthy foods
7. Prioritizing sleep
8. Writing
9. Watching funny movies and TV shows
10. Taking breaks from work
11. Singing and listening to beautiful music
12. Playing scrabbles and chess
13. Maintaining association or socialization
14. Avoiding sugary and highly processed food
15. Praying and meditation
16. Shopping
17. Cooking, baking
18. Ballroom dancing, aerobic dancing, weightlifting
19. Gardening, embroidery, cross stitching
20. Traveling
21. Hugging your loved one
22. Spending time with children, friends, and family
23. Pet an animal
24. Go to the museum.
25. Watch an opera or theater.

What do you think about these suggestions? What have you noticed?

Any activity that moves the body fosters good relationships, calms the nerves, and promotes well-being is good for the aging brain or brain. It is of the utmost importance to make time for worthwhile pursuits. Be kind to ourselves and mitigate stress.

Experiences throughout a person's lifetime can make him wise. Characters and relationship satisfaction are more defined. Aging may show a particular type of peace that cannot be seen among the young. These are the advantages of aging.

References:
1. https://www.ncbi.nlm.nih.gov/pmc/articles/PMC4906299/

Chapter 2
What is Dementia?
What is Alzheimer's disease?
Why Alzheimer's disease?

The entire world was shocked and saddened to know that the beloved Hollywood star Bruce Willis was diagnosed with Frontotemporal dementia. When his family shared this terrible ordeal in 2023, it garnered a slew of sympathy from his adoring fans. The following year, Wendy Williams, a famous Television talk show host, shared the same diagnosis. Her documentary was widely watched, and many people poured their love for her. In 2014, the world cried when Robin Williams, a comedian and versatile actor, committed suicide. Later, his wife admitted that he had been suffering from symptoms of Lewy body dementia, such as memory loss, personality changes, and sleep deprivation. Robin Williams felt there was no hope and resorted to suicide to end his dilemma.

Dementia does not choose anyone. It can affect a lowly servant and an Emperor. It knows no skin color, gender, race, and age. It has no mercy and no sympathy. It devours not only the person afflicted but their families as well. At worst, it can kill.

Other famous personalities that has had dementia or Alzheimer's disease are the following.
1. Charles Bronson, actor
2. Joanne Woodward, actress
3. Aaron Spelling, producer
4. Sean Connery, actor
5. Rita Hayworth, actress
6. Ronald Raegan, president
7. Rosa Parks, activist
8. Aaron Copland, composer
9. Perry Como, singer, actor, and TV personality

What is dementia?

How is it different from Alzheimer's disease?

Is it a normal part of aging?

Dementia and Alzheimer's Disease are often used interchangeably by most people; however, in a lot of sense, they are different. Dementia is an umbrella term for abnormal cognitive decline, impaired judgment, behavioral changes, and neuropsychiatric disorders. Alzheimer's is the most common cause of Dementia in the elderly. Dementia is not a normal part of aging and should not be mistaken for average age-related memory loss. People with dementia have lost their brain executive abilities such as problem-solving, language, and written comprehension and expression. These individuals may have impaired sound judgment, difficulty in day-to-day decision-making, inability to perform simple tasks such as self-care or sustenance, and inability to make financial decisions and choices. Coupled with impaired executive functioning, most people with dementia have behavioral problems such as agitation and depression. They may be socially isolated and, in some extreme forms, may suffer from delusions and or psychosis. People with dementia are reliant on their caregivers for their activities of daily living (ADL).

Dementia can be typified according to the part of the brain affected and the morphological changes in the cell or tissue. It is classified as Lewy body dementia, vascular dementia, frontotemporal dementia, or mixed dementia. Alzheimer's disease is the most common type of dementia in the elderly. Most Alzheimer's disease diagnoses are paired with vascular dementia, which has a graver prognosis.

My friend P.A.'s MRI result revealed two types of dementia: Alzheimer's disease and vascular dementia. This was confirmed by the presence of multiple ischemic strokes on various parts of her brain. P.A.'s medical history showed she suffered from hypertension and diabetes. Her diet was loaded with processed and sugary foods, too. She was sedentary, bound to her chair most of the day. Her faulty lifestyle predisposed her to chronic illnesses, which may have contributed to her dementia. It is essential to know that although stroke increases the risk of dementia, not all stroke patients will develop this dreadful illness.

Why are we interested in Alzheimer's disease?

What is the implication of this illness to a person and their immediate family?

When was Alzheimer's disease discovered?

Who uncovered this terrible illness?

In 1906, Dr. Alois Alzheimer was shocked to speak when a woman who was institutionalized had severe cognitive decline. Her name was Auguste Deter, a 50-year-old woman from Germany. During Dr. Alois's rounds and consultations, he would ask her simple questions such as her husband's name, current address, the weather, and her location. Ms. Deter was unable to answer. In addition, she also misnames objects and cannot recall her most recent memories. Ms. Deter's condition deteriorated. When she died, Dr. Alois performed an autopsy. He noticed that her brain was shrunk and had numerous plaques. He associated these abnormal findings with Ms. Deter's cognitive impairment and subsequent demise. Due to his efforts, this condition was named after him.

Many efforts have been made to identify the real cause of Alzheimer's disease. Scientists have concluded mechanisms as to its development. They have identified genetic problems and multifactorial causes that can increase the risk of its development. Pharmaceutical companies developed drugs to help stop its progression, but to no avail. To date, there is no cure for this dreadful condition.

References:

1. https://www.ninds.nih.gov/health-information/disorders/dementias
2. https://www.nia.nih.gov/health/alzheimers-and-dementia/alzheimers-disease-fact-sheet
3. https://www.nia.nih.gov/health/vascular-dementia/vascular-dementia-causes-symptoms-and-treatments
4. https://alzheimer.ca/en/about-dementia/what-alzheimers-disease/history-behind-alzheimers-disease

Alzheimer's Disease Basic Facts
1. Most common cause of dementia in older individuals.
2. Five million adults aged 65 and older are afflicted.
3. It is a neurodegenerative condition that develops gradually and is structurally characterized by neuronal cell death, loss of synaptic communication, the presence of extracellular plaques, and intra-neuronal tangles.
4. It affects memory, judgment, comprehension, behavior, language, executive functioning, and attention.
5. It has an early onset, manifested before age 65, and late-onset, which occurs after 65.
6. 5-10 percent is due to genetics, while 90 percent is multifactorial.
7. Diagnosis is based on history, signs and symptoms, MRI or other neuroimaging markers, such as amyloid and tau PET scans, and CSF and plasma markers, such as amyloid, tau, and phospho-tau levels.
   a. CT SCAN or volumetric MRI results reveal cerebral atrophy and a widened 3rd ventricle, with changes in the brain volume.
   b. PET, fMRI, and SPECT show a pattern of dysfunction in the brain.
   c. CSF analysis shows an increase in tau protein and a decrease in Beta amyloid 42.

    d. Neuropsychological test shows changes in memory, attention, language deficit, recall and retention, executive functioning problems, behavioral disorder, wandering, sleep disturbances, agitation, delusions, or psychosis.
8. Risk factors include obesity, diabetes, genetics, trisomy 21 or Down's syndrome, traumatic brain injury, depression, cerebrovascular disease, cardiovascular disease, smoking, family history, increased levels of homocysteine, presence of APOE, e4 allele, and advancing age.
9. Pathophysiological characteristics
    a. Abnormal extracellular amyloid plaques
    b. Intraneuronal fibrillary tangles
    c. Granulovacuolar degeneration of the hippocampal pyramidal cells
    d. Neuronal and synaptic losses
10. No treatment is available. Drugs such as cholinesterase inhibitors or NMDA antagonists are given to treat symptoms.
11. Quality of life could be better.

Individuals who have Alzheimer's are painful to see. I can personally tell you because of my friend P.A. She appeared confused most of the time. She has no recollection of the family she built or the friendships she fostered. She was consumed with so many delusions and anxiety. She became aggressive and demanding. In the end, she had to be institutionalized for her safety and those around her.

But the unsung heroes in these stories are the caregivers who care for them. This is a challenging task—caregivers Labor Day and night to meet the high demands of their work.

So, I asked my followers about their challenges while caring for their loved ones.

"It is so difficult. Some episodes are too hard to handle, and you cannot do anything but assist, care, and explain to them. The people who care for them should be patient and, more importantly, understanding."

Katherine Gamboa

"While busy washing the laundry, I left her in her wheelchair so she could get some sunshine. When I returned, I found her playing with her waste, putting it in her hair and saying it was a shampoo. She does not know me anymore, even though I was with her most of the time."

Alicia Bucawe

"My grandmother, who has dementia, would eat anything. She would also play with her feces. I asked her who I was, and she has no idea."

Emeleene Geolagon

"My dad, he passed away in May 2022. It came to a stage where he became incapacitated. He did not know how to eat, chew and swallow. He has forgotten how to speak, too."

Mellanie Endona Panesa Vergara

"My father would leave the house and ride a bus. The bus conductor would call us, saying he was already in Laguna. Another time, he was in Manila Police Station. It is good he still remembered our contact number. One time, a colleague saw him just wandering."

Mercy Viray Admana

Caregivers of patients with Alzheimer's disease may bear the brunt of the physical and emotional work. They may do this for years and often feel unsatisfied and unappreciated. Therefore, it is crucial to support them and, when possible, give them breaks and make room for relaxing activities. Here are some ways to care for their well-being while caring for their patients.

1. It is essential to ask for help when needed.
2. Eating healthy foods should be a priority. Nutritious foods give them energy.
3. Exercise can be a stress kicker.
4. Spend time with special people such as friends, family, and spouse.
5. Consider being a member of a support group.
6. Maintain a hobby.

Caregivers should always be kind to themselves. It is also essential to identify when they become burnt out, exhausted, upset, and irritated. Take a breather. Caregiving can be stressful, but it can also be rewarding. Everything is more accessible, knowing that you are not alone, and that help is always available.

References:

1. https://www.ncbi.nlm.nih.gov/books/NBK499922/
2. https://www.ninds.nih.gov/health-information/disorders/dementias
3. https://www.nia.nih.gov/health/alzheimers-caregiving/alzheimers-caregiving-caring-yourself

Chapter 3
Alternative Options for Alzheimer's Disease

There is no cure for Alzheimer's disease. The alternatives mentioned in this book are for educational use only. If you want to try them, we urge you to ask your medical professional. Some of these substances may affect other medications. The alternative options enumerated here may not be safe and can cause harm. We urge you to use discretion.

I.   Lithium

Drugs for Alzheimer's disease is developed based on Dr. Alois' discovery of abnormal plaques on the brain of Ms. Deter. Today, scientists have discovered more mechanisms for how dementia progresses, and based on these findings, they can formulate drugs to mitigate this condition. However, Alzheimer's disease is still incurable, and present medications are geared towards alleviation of symptoms.

A systematic review and meta-analysis of patients with Alzheimer's and Parkinson's disease revealed that lithium has reduced the amyloid-beta plaques and tau levels, and therefore, a noticeable improvement in cognition was observed in the animals' model. The analysis further confirms that lithium afforded some neuroprotection.

Studies by some scientists showed that lithium stabilizes disruptive calcium homeostasis, which helps modify the disease process in patients with Alzheimer's disease. Lithium was also shown to help improve neuroplasticity and cognitive function and slow down neuronal loss.

Agitation, aggression, and, in some severe cases, psychosis can accompany Alzheimer's disease. There is no FDA-approved drug for agitation among these patients. A randomized, double-blind, placebo control trial was done to assess how effective lithium is in the treatment of symptoms of agitation with or without psychosis in Alzheimer's disease. (I have attached the references if you want to read them more thoroughly.) There was a change in the aggression/agitation domain score, and neuropsychiatric symptoms improved after 12 weeks.

If you feel that lithium can help your loved one, it is crucial to talk to your medical professional. Lithium has some side effects and can affect how other drugs are metabolized in the body. Do not take lithium on your judgment. Ask your doctor for more information.

References:

1. https://pubmed.ncbi.nlm.nih.gov/38364914/
2. https://pubmed.ncbi.nlm.nih.gov/37666228/
3. https://www.ncbi.nlm.nih.gov/pmc/articles/PMC6082137/.

II.   Lion's Mane

Hericeum erinaceus is a functional food used in many recipes worldwide. It has a mild, sweet taste with a tender, chewable texture. It can be added to soups or sauteed with vegetables. Lion's mane can be a plant-based or vegetarian substitute for proteins such as poultry and beef. It is rich in fiber, beta-glucan, protein, carbohydrates, vitamins, and minerals. Several kinds of literature attest to the brain-health-promoting effects of Hericeum erinaceus; erinacine A, the active component, induces a neuroprotective factor. This substance increased the catecholamine content in the locus ceruleus and the hippocampus of rats in studies. Therefore, there was a marked improvement in the behavior and neuronal survival in different aspects of the brain. Erinacine A decreased beta-amyloid plaque formation and deposition.

References:

1. https://www.ncbi.nlm.nih.gov/pmc/articles/PMC5987239/
2. Shimbo M., Kawagishi H., Yokogoshi H. Erinacine A increases catecholamine and nerve growth factor content in the central nervous system of rats. *Nutrition Research.* 2005;**25**(6):617–623. doi: 10.1016/j.nutres.2005.06.001. [CrossRef] [Google Scholar] [Ref list]
3. Lee K. F., Chen J. H., Teng C. C., et al. Protective effects of *Hericium erinaceus* mycelium and its isolated erinacine A against ischemia-injury-induced neuronal cell death via inhibiting iNOS/p38 MAPK and nitrotyrosine. *International Journal of Molecular Sciences.* 2014;**15**(9):15073–15089. doi: 10.3390/ijms150915073. [PMC free article] [PubMed] [CrossRef] [Google Scholar] [Ref list]

III.   Short Chain Fatty Acids and Gut Microbiota

Multiple studies have focused on the ecology and health of gut microbiota. Healthy gut microbiota has been linked to numerous benefits, while an imbalance can cause problems. Short-chain fatty acids are the product of anaerobic fiber fermentation of probiotics. These substances exert physiological effects on their host, including immune, appetite regulation, and improved metabolism.

Research shows that alterations in the number, types, and health of gut microorganisms due to diet, antibiotic and drug intake, the presence of co-morbid conditions such as diabetes, and some lifestyle changes may contribute to the occurrence of multiple health problems, including Alzheimer's disease.

Transplantation of healthy gut microorganisms from healthy mice to those of mice with Alzheimer's disease was shown to help with their cognition and markedly reduce beta-amyloid plaque burden, inflammatory markers, and intraneuronal fibrillary tau proteins in their brains.

In addition to the ecological balance and health of the gut microbiota, the production of short-chain fatty acids from the anaerobic digestion of dietary fibers seemed to help mitigate the progression of Alzheimer's disease.

What is a short-chain fatty acid, and why are they so important?

Short-chain fatty acids are a type of saturated fat containing six carbons or less, are produced in the large intestines, and are effectively absorbed in the colonic epithelium. The most important SCFA are acetic, propionic, and butyric acid. SCFA, such as butyric acid, can cross the blood-brain barrier, exerting multiple effects on the central nervous system. This includes improvement in synaptic plasticity, communication, and brain cell development. It also reverses microglial damage and decreases neuroinflammation by reducing proinflammatory cytokines. SCFA interferes with beta-amyloid plaque formation and maintains the integrity of the blood-brain barrier.

References:

1. https://www.ncbi.nlm.nih.gov/pmc/articles/PMC9286902/
2. Qian XH, Song XX, Liu XL, Chen SD, Tang HD (2021). Inflammatory pathways in Alzheimer's disease mediated by gut microbiota. *Ageing Res Rev*, 68:101317. [PubMed] [Google Scholar] [Ref list]
3. Alexander C, Swanson KS, Fahey GC, Garleb KA (2019). Perspective: Physiologic Importance of Short-Chain Fatty Acids from Nondigestible Carbohydrate Fermentation. *Adv Nutr*, 10:576-589. [PMC free article] [PubMed] [Google Scholar] [Ref list]
4. McNeil NI, Cummings JH, James WP (1978). Short-chain fatty acid absorption by the human large intestine. *Gut*, 19:819-822. [PMC free article] [PubMed] [Google Scholar] [Ref list]

5. Dinan TG, Cryan JF (2017). Gut instincts: microbiota as a critical regulator of brain development, aging, and neurodegeneration. *J Physiol*, 595:489-503. [PMC free article] [PubMed] [Google Scholar] [Ref list]

IV.   Medium Chain Triglyceride (MCT)

Alzheimer's disease has been termed diabetes type 3 by numerous scientists because of impaired cerebral glucose and insulin metabolism. The brain relies heavily on sugar as its primary energy source using around 120 to 130 g/day. Failure to utilize sugar for food through cerebral insulin resistance, abnormal cerebral glucose metabolism, or anomalies in cerebral glucose receptors can result in cerebral atrophy, which is morphologically evident in the brains of Alzheimer's patients. These changes can significantly affect cognition, judgment, and behavior. MCT provides an alternative usable energy known as ketones, which are evident in blood circulation during fasting states when fats are burned. Ketones provide brain energy.

In a randomized, double-masked, placebo-controlled, cross-over study with an open-label extension, the use of MCT oil stabilized and improved the symptoms of Alzheimer's patients.

MCT oil is from coconut oil. Use coconut oil that is cold-pressed and unrefined.

References:
1. https://www.ncbi.nlm.nih.gov/pmc/articles/PMC8919247/
2. Owen OE, Morgan AP, Kemp HG, Sullivan JM, Herrera MG, Cahill GF. Brain metabolism during fasting. *J Clin Invest*. 1967;46:1589–1595. [PMC free article] [PubMed] [Google Scholar] [Ref list]

V.   Vitamins

Vitamins are organic substances derived from foods or made in vivo by the body, as in the case of Vitamin D. They are vital for health and act as cofactors in many enzymatic activities.

In Alzheimer's disease and most chronic illnesses, the production and accumulation of free radicals increase noticeably. These free radicals exert cellular damage and inflammation. Most vitamins act as free radical scavengers and antioxidants. They decrease lipid peroxidation, beta-amyloid deposition in the brain, and inflammation. Vitamins regulate cellular activities and metabolism and help maintain homeostasis.

A. B vitamins

B vitamins decrease the levels of homocysteine in the body. Its presence has been implicated in the development of several neurodegenerative disorders and cardiovascular risks. B12 is required for the conversion of homocysteine to methionine. Thus, deficiencies in B12, B6, and B9 can cause homocysteine accumulation in the body. In individuals with Alzheimer's disease, the Vitamin B12 level is typically low. It is, therefore, essential to supplement and nourish these individuals with Vitamin B12-rich foods such as meat, eggs, dairy products, and fish.

DNA methylation is usually impaired in Alzheimer's patients. Folate can assist in DNA methylation. In addition, inflammatory markers were lower among Alzheimer's patients who were given folic acid supplementation. Folates are usually found in green leafy vegetables.

B. Vitamin A

Vitamin A, or Beta carotene, is found in plants and is abundant in squash, pumpkins, tomatoes, carrots, and cantaloupe. Animal-derived Vitamin A, or retinol, is mainly seen in the liver and eggs. Vitamin A is essential for improved vision, normal cell differentiation, skin integrity, and strong immunity. It is also crucial in nerve cell maturation and proper neurotransmitter expressions for cell-to-cell communication.

Microglial hypo functioning has been noted in people with low Vitamin A. Microglial activation is associated with neuroinflammation and is typical in dementia.

Adding foods rich in Vitamin A to individuals with Alzheimer's may help improve their cognition.

C. Vitamin C and E

Seeds, nuts, avocados, and green leafy vegetables such as spinach are rich in vitamin E. Vitamin E is essential for reducing lipid peroxidation and beta-amyloid plaques.

Peppers, berries, cruciferous foods, citrus fruits, and potatoes are rich in vitamin C. Vitamin C acts as an antioxidant, free radical scavenger, and heavy metal chelator, thus reducing the inflammatory burden in people with dementia.

D. Vitamin D

Vitamin D is a fat-soluble vitamin that acts as a hormone in the body and is a potent antioxidant. It helps regulate calcium activity in the body, improves depression, and enhances immunity. Vitamin D is found in fatty fish and fortified foods. Sun exposure is the primary source of Vitamin D for most people.

An increase in cognitive impairment has been seen in individuals with lower levels of Vitamin D. Supplementation of Vitamin D may help improve behavior and mental cognition. Vitamin D mitigates neuroinflammation. It increases phagocytic activity in the brain, facilitating the removal of abnormal amyloid plaques. It can potentiate the effects of other drugs, thus increasing its neuroprotection.

References:

1. https://www.ncbi.nlm.nih.gov/pmc/articles/PMC7696081/
2. Smith P.J., Blumenthal J. Dietary Factors and Cognitive Decline. *J. Prev. Alzheimer Dis.* 2016;3:53–64. [PMC free article] [PubMed] [Google Scholar] [Ref list]
3. Chen H., Liu S., Ji L., Wu T., Ji Y., Zhou Y., Zheng M., Zhang M., Xu W., Huang G. Folic Acid Supplementation Mitigates Alzheimer's Disease by Reducing Inflammation: A Randomized Controlled Trial. *Mediat. Inflamm.* 2016;2016:1–10. doi: 10.1155/2016/5912146. [PMC free article] [PubMed] [CrossRef] [Google Scholar]
4. Wołoszynowska-Fraser M.U., Kouchmeshky A., McCaffery P. Vitamin A and Retinoic Acid in Cognition and Cognitive Disease. *Annu. Rev. Nutr.* 2020;40:247–272. doi: 10.1146/annurev-nutr-122319-034227. [PubMed] [CrossRef] [Google Scholar] [Ref list]
5. Sodhi R.K., Singh N. Retinoids as potential targets for Alzheimer's disease. *Pharmacol. Biochem. Behav.* 2014;120:117–123. doi: 10.1016/j.pbb.2014.02.016. [PubMed] [CrossRef] [Google Scholar] [Ref list]
6. Aguilar-Navarro S.G., Mimenza-Alvarado A.J., Jiménez-Castillo G.A., Bracho-Vela L.A., Yeverino-Castro S.G., Ávila-Funes J.A. Association of Vitamin D with Mild Cognitive Impairment and Alzheimer's Dementia in Older Mexican Adults. *Rev. Investig. Clin.* 2019;71:381–386. doi: 10.24875/ric.19003079. [PubMed] [CrossRef] [Google Scholar] [Ref list]
7. Annweiler C. Vitamin D in dementia prevention. *Ann. N. Y. Acad. Sci.* 2016;1367:57–63. doi: 10.1111/nyas.13058. [PubMed] [CrossRef] [Google Scholar] [Ref list]

VI.   Omega 3 fatty acids

It has been noted that a decreased intake of foods rich in Omega-3 fatty acids has been associated with an increased risk of cognitive decline or dementia. Omega 3 fatty acids are not only safe and inexpensive, but they are also protective of many chronic diseases. Chronic illnesses such as diabetes, hypertension, metabolic disease, and dyslipidemia have been shown to increase the risk of cognitive decline. Therefore, consuming foods high in this type can directly and indirectly affect the brain's health. Omega 3 fatty acid decreases neuroinflammation and reduction of amyloid plaques.

References:
1. https://www.ncbi.nlm.nih.gov/pmc/articles/PMC4019002/

VII.   Herbs
   1. Ashwagandha
   2. Brahmi
   3. Cat's claw
   4. Ginkgo biloba
   5. Saffron
   6. Turmeric

Ashwagandha has been used as a health tonic and is revered for its effect on longevity. Brahmi is recommended for alleviating stress, memory lapses, seizures, and insomnia. Ginkgo biloba is utilized as a memory enhancer, while Gotu Kola has been noted to help promote intelligence and memory.

In vitro, in vivo, and clinical studies suggest these herbs have neuroprotective effects. They are potent antioxidants and free radical scavengers. They exert anti-inflammatory properties. These herbs also prevented neuronal demise, which helped mitigate cognitive decline. They restored synaptic activity, thus improving cell-to-cell communication. They helped in neuronal regeneration, enhanced neurotransmitter content and action, and decreased beta-amyloid deposition.

Herbs may carry risks, so you must ask your medical health professional before adding plants to your daily routine.

References:
1. https://www.ncbi.nlm.nih.gov/pmc/articles/PMC8068256/

2. Howes M.J., Houghton P.J. Plants are used in Chinese and Indian traditional medicine to improve memory and cognitive function. *Pharmacol. Biochem. Behav.* 2003;75:513–527. doi: 10.1016/S0091-3057(03)00128-X. [PubMed] [CrossRef] [Google Scholar] [Ref list]

Chapter 4
Other Factors to Consider

1. Estrogen and Alzheimer's disease

Estrogen is a hormone that has numerous health implications for the female gender, which includes protection from heart disease, osteopenia, or osteoarthritis and as an antioxidant.

Alzheimer's disease, which is common among women, indicates that estrogen deficiency may be a risk factor. Research has shown that estrogen may be protective by reducing neural inflammation, increasing cholinergic and serotonergic activities, and reducing damage by free radicals.

References:
https://www.ncbi.nlm.nih.gov/pmc/articles/PMC10480684/

2. Air pollution and Alzheimer's disease

Pollution contributes to many modern diseases, such as cancer, respiratory disorders such as asthma, and infectious and degenerative illnesses.

Exposure to air pollutants or particulate matter is a risk factor for the development of dementia. These toxic pollutants can enter the body and lodge in the brain, causing damage. The direct damage can lead to symptoms of Alzheimer's disease.

References:
https://www.nih.gov/news-events/nih-research-matters/air-pollution-linked-dementia-cases

3. Malnutrition and Alzheimer's disease

Nutrition is an essential aspect of a person's life. In every stage of human development, their nutritional requirements change. For the young and old, pregnant and nursing, in cases of stress, trauma, or burns, the requirement increases. Males have different needs compared to females.

Nutritional problems differ in different parts of the world. In America, where food is abundant, obesity is alarmingly increasing. However, in some parts of Africa, children are dying of starvation every day. As some countries abandon their traditional ways of consuming food and welcome the Western diet that is high in processed, sugary, and oily food, most people have developed chronic illnesses that are associated with their consumption. Diet, especially a proper diet rich in complex carbohydrates and fiber, healthy fats such as seeds and nuts, fruits, and vegetables have been shown to promote health and longevity.

Individuals with Alzheimer's often complain of loss of appetite. This dilemma can lead to weight loss and subsequent malnutrition. When nutritional status is severely compromised, cognitive decline worsens. In addition, behavioral and psychological problems such as aggression, depression, and psychosis may occur. To correct this problem, the patient may require hospitalization or intensive care. In some cases, individuals with Alzheimer's may be permanently institutionalized.

References:
https://www.ncbi.nlm.nih.gov/pmc/articles/PMC6723872/

4. Metals and Alzheimer's disease
Heavy metals and toxins such as mercury, cadmium, arsenic, aluminum, and lead are some of the leading causes of illnesses in humanity. They exert biological activity in the cell, disrupting its normal enzymatic activities. They can cause problems in protein formation and processing, causing misfolding, abnormal aggregation, and phosphorylation. They can attack DNA and influence gene expression. As some can cross the blood-brain barrier, they can damage the brain's delicate architecture, leading to alterations in intelligence and behavior.

Particulate matter in the air may contain heavy metals such as lead, cadmium, and manganese; these neurotoxins may increase the risk for Alzheimer's disease and dementia as they can cause direct and indirect damage to the brain. In some epidemiologic studies, these heavy metals have been associated with mental decline.

Heavy metals are usually present in paints, gasoline, soil, plumbing, fertilizers, mining, and fossil fuels.

References:
https://www.ncbi.nlm.nih.gov/pmc/articles/PMC7454042/

5. Infection and Alzheimer's disease
Infectious diseases can predispose a person to develop a more severe condition. Chronic Hepatitis B can increase the risk of hepatocellular carcinoma. Epstein Barr Virus has been implicated in nasal carcinoma,

while schistosomiasis may cause transitional cell carcinoma of the urinary bladder. Human papillomavirus may cause cervical cancer.

Viral encephalitis from a virus has been linked to the development of Alzheimer's disease. A person is 30 times more likely to be diagnosed with Alzheimer's disease than those who have none.

References:
https://www.nih.gov/news-events/nih-research-matters/links-found-between-viruses-neurodegenerative-diseases

Chapter 5
Closer Look at Alzheimer's Disease

A. Sundowning

People with Alzheimer's are usually more agitated, depressed, or aggressive at a particular time of the day. This phenomenon is called sundowning, in which neuropsychiatric symptoms usually happen or worsen. External or internal factors can trigger it, or it can occur spontaneously. Affected individuals would scream, fight, wander, or would succumb to delusions and hallucinations. Sundowning can affect their sleep and eating patterns. There is no definitive causative factor to explain why Alzheimer's patients act in this manner. There is no precise management or drug regimen for this bizarre occurrence. Being aware, familiar, and expectant of this phenomenon would help the caregivers and their families to overcome this challenge.

A wandering patient should be secured. If possible, alarms should be installed in the room. It is crucial to put a fixed bracelet on their arms containing important information such as their name, address, and telephone number.

For people with anxiety and aggressive tendencies, an anti-anxiety pill may help.

Reference:
https://www.ncbi.nlm.nih.gov/pmc/articles/PMC5187352/

B. Time Distortions

The ability to perceive, identify, and rationalize time is essential to human functioning. Time perception affects behavior, cognition, judgment, and executive functions. Timing is required to act on a problem. Time recognition tells us if it is time to sleep or be alert. Time also tells us when to eat or not. Time perception is empirical to human survival.

Time perception is flawed among Alzheimer's patients. The loss of the ability to tell and use time is due to abnormalities found in the hippocampal areas, which are also the seat for recall and memory. Symptoms such as insomnia or hypersomnia, confusion, inability to discern the exact time of the day, dates, and months, and overlapping of old and new memories are attributed to this dysfunction.

Reference:
https://www.ncbi.nlm.nih.gov/pmc/articles/PMC5514999/

Chapter 6
Doctor Farrah Protocol

The 5 Facets of the Doctor Farrah Protocol

My journey in Medicine has been filled with many inaccuracies and fallacies. I used to believe that the typical diet is enough to sustain a person's nutritional requirements. Therefore, supplementation with vitamins and minerals is not only a waste of time but also a waste of resources. I used to believe that mega-dosing in vitamins and minerals is detrimental to health. Plants have no healing properties and do not exert any physiologic activities in the body. I used to think that the consumption of herbs may harm the kidneys and the liver. I used to believe that maintenance drugs are crucial to health. An aspirin may halt a heart attack; a statin lowers total cholesterol; these drugs are effective and safe. Hypertension and Diabetes are incurable, as I was taught in school. I was taught fluoride is necessary to reduce dental caries and strong teeth. I used to believe that high Cholesterol and saturated fats are bad and are the leading cause of atherosclerosis and, thus, heart and brain stroke. My teachers did not caution me about radiation; instead, they reassured me that numerous chest X-rays in a year are safe. I used to believe that vaccines offer substantial protection against a disease.

Medical schools only teach the most essential part of medicine. Most of them must be discovered through continuous education and research. Medical education is pharmacologically driven, ignoring or putting little emphasis on the importance of natural medicine and nutritional science. Most medical procedures performed in the hospital have no solid science behind them. Diagnosis is mainly intelligent guesswork. Most physicians don't know what they are doing. They disagree most of the time. A second or even third opinion is crucial to arrive at a correct diagnosis and treatment. A patient-related his experience in the hospital after suffering from severe diarrhea. Since he also had diabetes, hypertension, and heart disease, four doctors were assigned to oversee him. In the end, he left the hospital with tons of bills and no improvement.

Dissatisfied with the standard of care and flawed medical system, natural medicine has given me a brighter hope and a chance to help the sick. Current research and studies have proven that plants have phytochemicals that can physiologically affect the person. These phytochemicals are safe, effective, and, in most instances, fast-acting. Lifestyle and diet modification, exercise, and environmental changes can offer numerous health benefits. In some cases, it is even better than what synthetic drugs can offer. With the expensive cost of the current medical system, natural medicine offers a cheaper alternative.

In the 20 years I have been a physician, I discovered that most illnesses are due to faulty diet, lifestyle, and exposure to environmental pollutants. The interplay of these factors is a recipe for disaster. Genetics plays a minor role in disease development. These genes can be turned on or off with proper nutrition. I concluded that in addition to correcting these faulty factors, faulty thinking should also be considered. Stress, hopelessness, and pessimism should be avoided.

Malnutrition is a significant source of problems for humanity. In America, where food is abundant, obesity is at a high level. In some countries where the staple food is white rice, they may be deficient in some vitamins. In Africa, where children die every day due to starvation, protein-calorie malnutrition is ravaging. Many factors affect malnutrition, initially from agricultural practices observed in that area. Farmers do not properly fertilize the soil anymore; they use chemical fertilizers, excessive pesticides, and herbicides. Processing vegetables and fruits and exposing them to oxidants decreases the vitamin content of these produce. Processing food, removing fibers, vitamins, and minerals, and adding excessive sugar to prolong shelf life have contributed to chronic diseases.

Malnutrition can happen when malabsorption conditions exist in a person. This includes a history of gut surgery, leaky gut, and diseases affecting the gastrointestinal tract. Age can also contribute to the level of malnutrition. Older adults and infants are more prone to symptoms of malnutrition.

Infection or infestation can cause significant health problems. In 3rd world countries, worms devastate children and adults and can cause anemia, nutritional issues, obstructive disorders, and, in extreme cases, behavioral problems. Human Papilloma Virus may cause the deadly cervical cancer among women. Hepatitis B and C are prone among drug users and is a sexually transmitted disease. Chronic infection with these viruses can increase the incidence of hepatocellular carcinoma. Viruses are self-limiting infections. The body must rely on a robust immune system to rid itself of it.

Toxins or heavy metals have been associated not only with cancer and autoimmune disease but, more importantly, with dementia. The toxins can come from occupational or environmental exposures. These toxins can cross the blood-brain barrier and cause damage to the brain. They can be deposited in the fat tissues for years and released into the circulation as they are burned.

The DRF protocol revolves around correcting malnutrition and removing infection, infestation, and toxins. I achieve this goal through the following,

    a. Vitamin-Mineral Therapy
    b. Herbal Therapy
    c. Nutritional Therapy
    d. Lifestyle and Environmental modification.

A. Vitamin-Mineral Therapy

Vitamins are organic substances that sustain and maintain life. Most vitamins are supplied in food. Vitamin D is produced in vivo through skin exposure to sunlight. These organic substances, such as Vitamin C, exert physiologic activities in the body. This vitamin is essential in producing collagen, strong immunity, and alleviating stress. Vitamin B is vital for skin integrity, proper blood cell production and maturation, brain health, enhanced energy, immune fortification, and effective digestion. Vitamin A is essential for healthy vision, beautiful skin, functioning immune cells, and cellular differentiation. Vitamin D is vital in healing depression and absorption of calcium in the intestinal mucosa. Vitamin E is good for heart health and protection from damage to the red blood cells, while Vitamin K is for proper blood clotting.

Minerals are inorganic substances found in the soil, air, and water. They are often called dusts of the soil or elements of nutrition. Minerals are essential because they are necessary for the body's metabolic or enzymatic activities. The body cannot create them, so diet must supply them. Minerals are not made in a vacuum, so the soil must be replenished through sensible organic farming.

Most illnesses are a result of mineral deficiencies or toxicities. Cadmium toxicity can result in hypertension and kidney and lung problems. Chromium deficiencies may lead to diabetes and atherosclerosis. Magnesium deficiencies have been associated with leukemias and lymphomas, seizures, depression, heart diseases, and sleep disturbances. Mercury and Aluminum toxicities have been shown to contribute to the formation of Alzheimer's, Parkinson's disease, dementia, mental retardation among infants, and some forms of cancers. Zinc deficiencies can cause problems in the immune system, obesity, acne, and infertility. Manganese deficiency can cause bone problems, depression, and even schizophrenia. Iodine deficiency can lead to obesity, menstrual problems, mental dullness, and infertility. Cobalt and Iron deficiencies can be seen as anemia and immune deficiencies. Excess sodium can cause seizures, while excess potassium in the circulation, especially in renal failure, can cause arrhythmia and subsequent death.

B. Herbal Therapy

The majority of pharmaceutical drugs in the market are derived from plants. Plant medicine, or Ethnobotany, is an exact, tested, and accurate science proven to exert physiologic effects on the body. Plants have phytochemicals such as lycopene, flavonoids, alkaloids, essential oils, and beta-glucans. In addition, they are rich in minerals, fibers, and vitamins. These phytochemicals act as anti-inflammatory, anti-microbial, anti-cancer, and antioxidant properties.

Guava leaves have anti-septic and anti-diarrheal properties. Oregano, chili peppers, and garlic have antibacterial properties. Eucalyptus soothes the bronchial lining. Lemon has skin-bleaching properties. Dandelion, burdock, and milk thistle protect the liver. Carrots can contribute to clearer eyesight. Honey and cinnamon are good for ridding cough and treating burns and skin blemishes. They have potent anti-inflammatory and anti-microbial properties. Coconut oil is valued for its conditioning effect on the skin, hair, and nails. Grapes have antiaging properties. Malabar spinach is excellent for the prevention and treatment of constipation. Horsetail, lemongrass, and stinging nettle are good for kidney problems such as infections and stones. Ginger may help calm an upset stomach. The active component gingerol proves to be an effective pain reliever. Chili pepper can help relieve pain if applied topically.

Plants can be boiled, steamed, juiced, or eaten raw. Tree barks should be boiled for 15 minutes, a procedure known as decoction. Stems, leaves, and flowers may be steeped in hot water for 5 minutes and then drunk. Tincture is usually done with alcohol or vodka.

The key to their efficacy depends on the herb's quantity and quality. Plants harvested for their medicinal properties should be grown in optimum conditions. The soil should be free from environmental contamination by lead, mercury, and cadmium. It should also be rich in minerals and organic substances and host numerous beneficial bacteria and other essential microscopic organisms.

As a rule, herbal use of plants is typically 5 or 7 handfuls. People should consume as many as they can. It does not make sense for someone to prepare a tea of 10 chili peppers if they can't drink it. Start from the lowest tolerable dose and then increase from that.

C. Nutritional Therapy

Nutrition is universal in Natural Medicine. Without proper food intake, metabolism, and assimilation, we are all bound to be sick, and if not corrected, this can lead to death.

Cancer loves processed sugar. It is vital to exclude processed sugar from the diet, both natural and synthetic. I believe that sweet fruits should not be given to cancer patients. Unripe fruits are exemptions. Simple carbohydrates or those easily converted to sugar in the body, such as white rice, white pasta, white bread, and potato, should be limited. I discourage the consumption of GMOs or genetically modified organisms. Our body does not have the enzymes to process these foods. Our body may react to these substances, causing an allergic reaction or inflammation. Inflammation is the basis of most chronic diseases, including cancer, metabolic disorders, and autoimmune diseases.

Processed foods like bacon, sausage, and hot dogs have nitrates. The nitrates prolong the shelf life of these foods. Nitrates have been proven to cause stomach cancer in numerous studies. Processed foods may also contain dyes that can cause inflammation. Currently, there are nine artificial dyes that USFDA approves that are likely to cause cancer, hypersensitivity, and behavioral problems. Synthetic dyes are derived from petroleum and enhance the color of foods. Yellow 5 and 6 and Red 40 particularly have benzidine, a known human and animal carcinogen. Artificial flavorings are also harmful to our health if consumed.

MSG, or Monosodium glutamate, has excitatory effects on the neuronal firings of the brain. This action may trigger headaches and seizures. In a study involving rat pups, the administration of MSG showed altered behavioral characteristics, tonic-clonic seizures, and electroencephalographic pattern alterations.

Aspartame or artificial sweeteners may be converted to wood alcohol and formaldehyde. Consuming these sugar substitutes has been shown to cause brain problems.

All canned foods should not be consumed. Canning is a method of preservation. The foods are usually processed and sealed in an airtight container. Some canned foods can last five years or more, provided the container has no leaks. The Bisphenol A from the can may leach and contaminate the food. Forty percent of studied canned goods have BPA on them. BPA is an endocrine disruptor that has been linked to the formation of numerous congenital disabilities and cancer. Also, some deadly bacteria may survive the heating method used to sterilize the food.

An example of this is Botulism, which can cause a rare but serious foodborne illness. Botulism can cause neurologic symptoms such as double vision and difficulty breathing and swallowing. Clostridium botulinum makes a lethal neurotoxin that can cause paralysis and even death.

As a rule, anything made by humans is harmful to our health. This includes cakes, candies, bread, and soft drinks. Therefore, whole foods such as unripe fruits, vegetables, nuts, fish, organic eggs, and organic meats are encouraged.

Organic means non-GMO has no growth hormones, no antibiotics, is vaccine-free, and is grass-fed.

Antibiotics are commonly used in growing animals to stop the growth of harmful bacteria that can kill the animals or harm consumers. However, antibiotics introduced to chickens, pigs, and cows can also be absorbed by humans when eaten. This influences the gut microbiota ecology and health. In addition, antibiotic resistance can happen consequently.

Growth hormones and steroids are usually injected into animals to increase their muscle mass. The introduction of exogenous hormones may upset the animals' homeostasis, and when consumed by humans, they may also affect their hormones. Excess exogenous hormones can give rise to cancer of reproductive organs.

Vaccines may contain harmful substances such as aluminum, formaldehyde, dyes, fetal cells, and mercury. When introduced into the animal and consumed, these substances may be passed on to the unsuspecting consumer and cause problems.

GMO corn and soya are usually fed to animals. These products can influence the health of these animals and, subsequently, the health of their consumers.

The cooking and processing of food reduces its vitamin and mineral content. Even the mere peeling of fruits eliminates essential vitamins such as Vitamin C and Vitamin B.

D. Lifestyle and Environmental Modification

Man has changed his environment for the worse. Mining, deforestation, and industrialization have caused the emergence of toxic and environmental pollutants in the air and water we drink.

Mercury poisoning was found on Japan's riverbank; the fish the people ate made them sick. The infants from the pregnant women who ate the contaminated fish developed severe mental retardation. Lead that is discharged from the exhaust to the air has contaminated the grasses, soil, water, and atmosphere. Cows who ate from them died. Paints may contain lead, mercury, benzene, or toluene. Benzene can cause liver and blood cancer. Formaldehyde, a binding agent in cheap furniture, can evaporate when heated. This can cause severe respiratory health problems to the occupants of the home.

Health and personal care products, household cleaning agents, and aerosol sprays are also laced with toxic substances we inhale, absorb, and expose ourselves to. Dyes and synthetic perfumes can cause allergic reactions, leading to eczema, dermatitis, and skin asthma. Strong deodorants may contain aluminum as a drying agent. Aluminum is a neurotoxin and a carcinogen.

Cooking utensils such as aluminum and Teflon should not be used. Cooking with refined, bleached, and deodorized oils, notably, has contributed to developing some diseases, such as cancer.

Exercising improves the body's overall function. Moving enhances brain function, immunity, bowel movement, kidney excretion, lymphatic drainage, and heart function.

Alcohol consumption is toxic to the liver and brain. Excessive alcohol intake can damage the liver and may result in cirrhosis or liver cancer.

Tobacco smoke is not only addictive but has contributed to numerous deaths around the world due to chronic obstructive pulmonary disease and an increased risk of cancer development in the oropharynx, lung, reproductive, and bladder.

Viral diseases like Hepatitis B, C, and D may lead to liver cancer. HPV is a causative factor in the formation of cervical cancer. HIV may cause Kaposi's sarcoma. Epstein Barr Virus has been demonstrated to cause nasopharyngeal carcinoma and lymphoma.

Parasitic infections like schistosomiasis can cause bladder and liver cancer. Toxoplasmosis can cause schizophrenia and congenital disease in unborn infants.

The Principles behind the Doctor Farrah Protocol

The human body is like a house. When we bring groceries and produce but do not take out the garbage or clean, the house will become congested and may stink. If the plumbing is obstructed and not cleared out, it will flood. This flooding can eventually destroy the house. If the septic is total overflows, it will devastate the home and the lawn.

Our body is simple. It is made up of different cells. Each cell is capable of eating and assimilation of nutrients. They can create proteins to carry out the functions needed for daily activities. The products of these activities can produce waste substances and must be excreted. When the cells become too old, they die in a process known as apoptosis or programmed cell death.

The world is organized, and the human body has extensive organization. Groups of cells make up tissues, and these tissues make up the organ. A group of organs comprises a system, including an individual. When there is a disruption in the balance and function within these systems, problems may arise. Problems may occur due to toxin overload, micronutrient and macronutrient deficiency, homeostatic imbalance, stress, sedentary lifestyle, and faulty lifestyle.

Let's talk about Alzheimer's disease. Alzheimer's disease happens because of genetics, but the majority happens because of multifactorial conditions. The brain shrinks with noticeable abnormal depositions of abnormal amyloid proteins and tau proteins inside the neurons. There is also a loss in synaptic communication and neuronal death. As a result, cognitive declines such as memory loss, impaired judgment, behavioral abnormalities, and failure to perform activities of daily life happen. There is no current treatment for Alzheimer's disease, and the drugs given to them are to slow down the occurrence or severance of the symptoms.

My protocol for Alzheimer's disease centers on proper nutrition, correction of micronutrient deficiency, and establishing support.

A. Herbal Remedies

Ingredients:
1. Turmeric
2. Pepper
3. Coconut Oil/milk

Boil two cups of water. Add crushed turmeric and a pinch of black pepper. Add ½ cups of coconut milk or 1 tbsp of coconut oil. Drink three times a day.

B. Micronutrient/Macronutrient Remedies
1. Phospholipid with butyric acid: 1 tsp 3x a day
2. Bile salts/acids: 1 capsule 3x a day
3. Boston C/Megadose Vitamin C/Pixie Dust Magnesium: 1 tsp each 3x a day

C. Nutritional Remedies

Avoid eating processed and sugary foods. Eat a plant-based diet high in protein, complex carbohydrates, fiber, and healthy fats. Consume small fatty fish, eggs, preferably organic, and nuts and seeds.

Caring for people with Alzheimer's disease is challenging. A strong and stable support system is essential to have.